The Effortless

Based Breakfast

Quick and Easy Plant-Based Recipes to Boost Your Breakfast and Improve Your Health

Carl Brady

Table of contents

Enriching Oatmeal Strawberry Smoothie

Preparation time: 5 minutes Cooking time: 0 minutes 2 servings.

Ingredients

14 strawberries

1 ½ cups soy milk

1 tsp. vanilla

1 banana

¼ cup oats

1 tsp. sugar

Directions:

Begin by bringing all the ingredients together in a blender and blending the ingredients to achieve desired consistency. Enjoy!

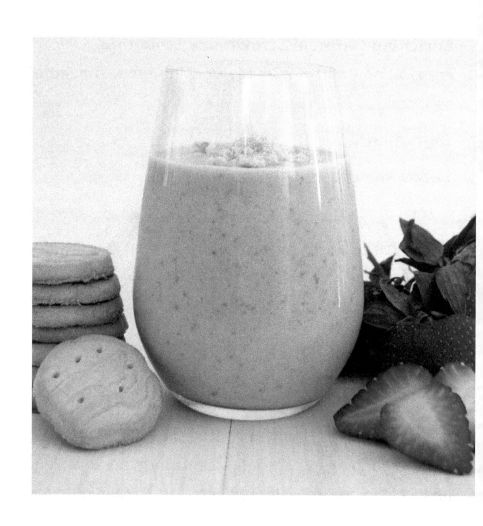

Scrambled Eggs with Spinach

Preparation Time: 5 minutes Cooking Time: 4 minutes
Servings: 2

Ingredients:

2 tsp. olive oil

3 cups baby spinach

4 eggs, beaten

Salt and pepper to taste

2 slices whole-wheat bread, toasted

1 cup raspberries, sliced

Direction:

Pour the olive oil into a pan over medium heat. Cook the spinach for 2 minutes. Transfer to a plate. Add the eggs to the pan. Cook while stirring frequently for 2 minutes. Add the spinach and season with salt and pepper. Serve scrambled egg on top of the bread, and with raspberries.

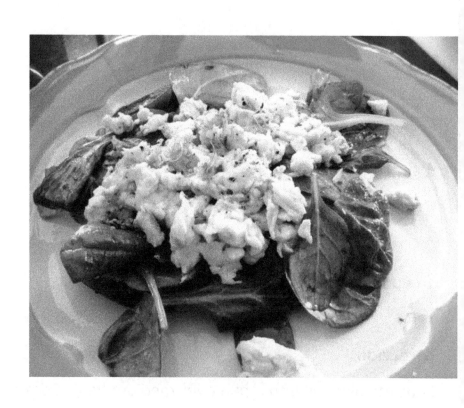

Protein Pancakes

Servings: 4 Preparation Time: 35 min

Ingredients:

1 scoop vegan protein powder

¼ cup almond flour

1 tbsp. glucomannan powder

1 ½ cup water

1 tbsp. flaxseed oil

1 tsp. vanilla extract

1 tsp. baking powder

Directions:

Soak glucomannan powder in ½ cup water for a couple of minutes. Combine all dry Ingredients and set aside. Mix vanilla extract and flaxseed oil with soaked glucomannan. Put a nonstick pan on the stove over medium heat. Slowly stir a cup of water into the dry flour mixture, and combine thoroughly. Add the glucomannan into flour and protein mixture. Stir well. Add heap of batter to the pan and spread out into a ¼ inch thick pancake. Bake for 5 minutes on each side and repeat this for all pancakes. Can be stored in fridge for 3 days or frozen for up to 2 months.

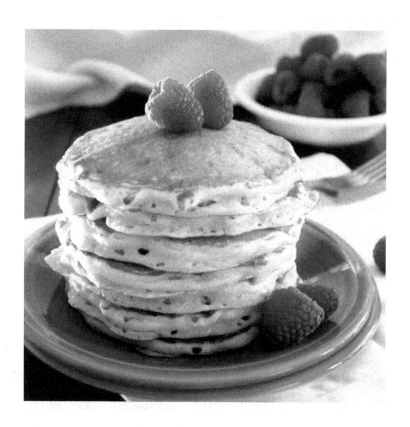

Spiced Pumpkin Oats

Preparation Time:10 minutes Cooking time:6 minutes Servings:1 Servings: 4

Ingredients

1 apple, peeled and grated

1 teaspoon vanilla extract

1 cup steel cut oats

¼ teaspoon ground cloves

¼ teaspoon ground nutmeg

1 teaspoon ground cinnamon

1 cup pumpkin puree

3 cups water After cooking

2 tablespoons pumpkin seeds

2 tablespoons maple syrup

Directions:

Combine the oats, water, grated apple, vanilla extract, cloves, nutmeg, cinnamon and pumpkin puree in a medium pot. Cover and bring the pot to a boil, lower the heat and simmer for around 25 minutes. Stir in the maple syrup, let it cool and then apportion into containers. To reheat, simply add a little almond milk and reheat in 30-second increments in the microwave until nice and hot. You can add additional maple syrup if you like.

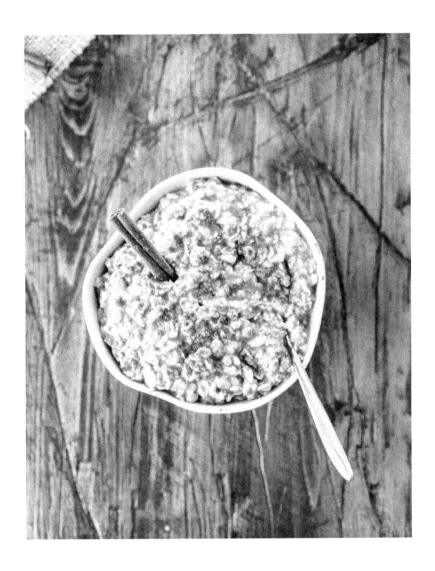

Sausage-wrapped Eggs

Preparation time: 5 minutes Cooking time: 40 minutes

Servings: 3

Ingredients:

1 egg, lightly beaten

6 hard-cooked eggs, peeled

1 pound Pork Sausage Roll

Salt Pepper

3/4 cup cornflakes, crushed

Directions:

Divide the sausage roll into six portions and then flatten. Season each portion with salt and pepper to taste. Shape each sausage portion around an egg. Roll in lightly beaten egg, and then in the cornflake crumbs. Place sausage-wrapped eggs on a rack placed in a baking pan and then bake, uncovered, at a temperature of 400° F for about half an hour minutes or until the meat no longer looks pink, turning eggs every 10 minutes.

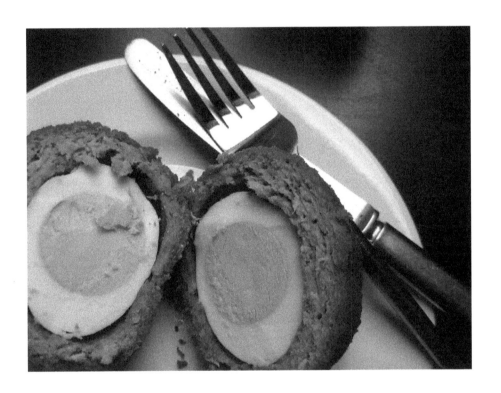

Egg Rolls

Preparation time: 5 minutes Cooking time: 20 minutes

Servings: 3

Ingredients:

1 -inch ginger, freshly grated

4 tablespoons of vegetable oil

2 cloves of garlic, finely chopped

10 cooked shrimps, minced

1 carrot, medium, cut into 1-inch strips (julienne)

2 green onion, sliced thinly

1 red pepper, small, cut into 1-inch strips (julienne)

1/4 cup of chicken broth

1 cup of shredded Napa cabbage

2 tablespoons of soy sauce, reduced-sodium variety

1 to 2 tablespoons of sesame oil

1 tablespoon of sugar

20 wonton wrappers, loosely covered with damp paper towel

Directions:

In a skillet or wok, heat 2 tablespoons of oil and stir-fry garlic and ginger until fragrant, which should take about 30 seconds. Add carrots, red pepper, and green onions. Over high heat, stir-fry for about 2 minutes. Combine the soy sauce, sugar, and chicken broth in a bowl. Then, add in the broth mixture and Napa cabbage into the pan. Bring to a just a rolling boil and then simmer about 5 minutes, while stirring occasionally, until vegetables are tender. Add the sesame oil, and allow to cool for a minimum of 15 minutes. Strain, and then fold in the shrimp. Fill the egg roll wrappers, using 1 a tablespoon of the cabbage-shrimp filling for each one. Work with a wonton wrapper at a time, positioning the wrapper in such a way that there is one corner of a diamond close to you. Put a teaspoon of filling in the center and then roll the corner of the wrapper closest to you, going over the cabbage-shrimp filling. Then, brush the wrapper's top corner using water and then fold in the wrapper's sides. Rolling up the wrapper with the filling until closed and then press to seal. Set finished roll aside, and do the same with remaining ingredients. In a pan set, heat remaining oil over moderately high heat and then sauté egg rolls until they become golden brown on all the sides. Use tongs to turn the rolls. When done, set on a plate and then serve when cool enough. This can be served with dipping sauce.

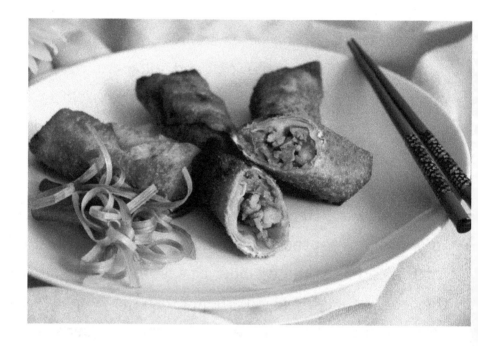

Vegan Breakfast Biscuits

Preparation Time: 10 minutes Cooking Time: 10 min Servings: 6

Ingredients:

cups Almond Flour

1 tbsp Baking Powder

¼ tsp Salt

½ tsp Onion Powder

½ cup Coconut Milk

¼ cup Nutritional Yeast

2 tbsp Ground Flax Seeds

¼ cup Olive Oil

Directions:

Preheat oven to 450F. Whisk together all Ingredients in a bowl. Divide the batter into a pre-greased muffin tin. Bake for 10 minutes.

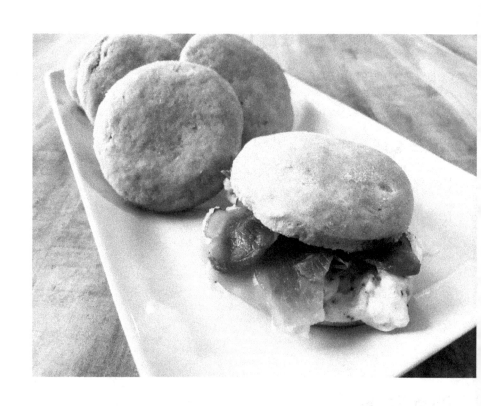

Vegan Breakfast Sausages

Preparation Time: 15 minutes Cooking Time: 12 min

Servings: 4

Ingredients:

200 grams Portobella Mushrooms

150 grams Walnuts 1 tbsp Tomato Paste

75 grams Panko

1 tsp Paprika

1 tsp Dried Sage

1 tsp Salt ½ tsp

Black Pepper

Directions:

Blend all Ingredients in a food processor. Divide mixture into serving-sized portions and shape into sausages. Bake for 12 minutes at 375F.

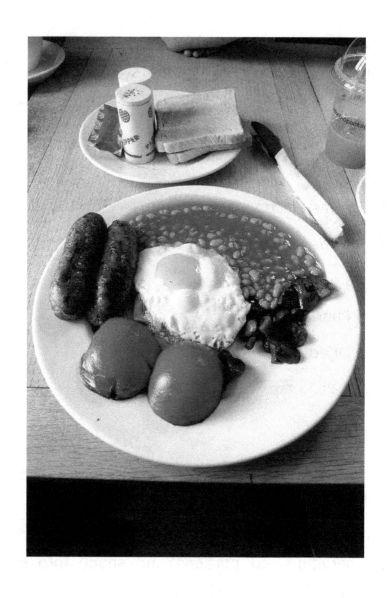

Spiced Tofu And Broccoli Scramble

Preparation Time: 5 minutes Cooking Time: 3 minutes

Servings: 3

Ingredients:

400 grams Firm Tofu, drained and pressed

1 tbsp Tamari

1 tbsp Garlic Powder

2 tsp Paprika Powder

2 tsp Turmeric Powder

150 grams Broccoli, rough-chopped

2 tbsp Olive Oil

Directions:

Crumble the tofu in a bowl with the garlic powder, paprika, turmeric, and nutritional yeast. Heat olive oil in a pan. Sautee broccoli for a minute. Stir in spiced tofu. Cook for 1-2 minutes. Season with tamari. Serve hot.

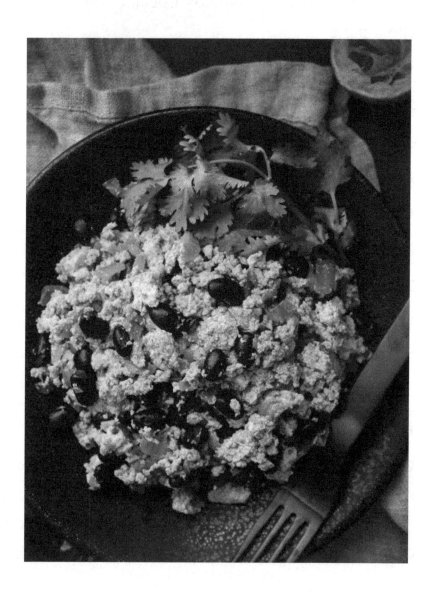

Vegan Southwestern Breakfast

Preparation Time: 10 minutes Cooking Time: 5 minutes

Servings: 6

Ingredients:

1 small White Onion, diced

1 Bell Pepper, diced

150 grams Mushrooms, sliced

400 grams Firm Tofu, crumbled

1 tsp Turmeric Powder

1 tbsp Garlic Powder

2 tbsp Nutritional Yeast

¼ cup Chopped Green Onions

2 cups Fresh Spinach

1 cup Cherry Tomatoes

2 cups Baked Beans

2 tbsp Olive Oil

Directions:

Sautee onions, bell peppers, and mushrooms until onions are translucent. Add in the tofu. Stir in the turmeric, garlic powder, and nutritional yeast. Add green onions and spinach. Sautee for 1-2 minutes. Serve with baked beans and cherry tomatoes.

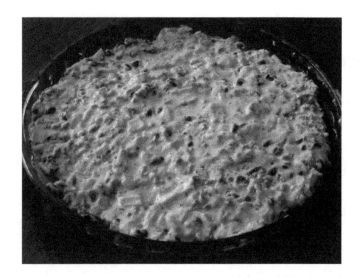

Kale Breakfast Sandwich

Preparation Time: 10 minutes Cooking time: 6 minutes

Servings: 1

Ingredients:

A drizzle of olive oil

2 cups kale, torn

A pinch of salt and black pepper

2 tablespoons pumpkin seeds

1 small shallot, chopped

½ teaspoon jalapeno, dried and crushed

1 and ½ tablespoons avocado mayonnaise

1 avocado slice

1 vegan bun, halved

Directions:

Heat up your air fryer with the oil at 360 degrees F, add kale, salt, pepper, pumpkin seeds, shallot and jalapeno, toss, cover and cook for 6 minutes shaking once. Spread avocado mayo on each muffin half, add the avocado slice, add the kale mix, top with the other muffin half and serve for breakfast. Enjoy!

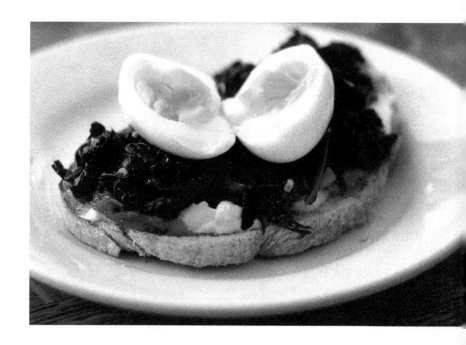

Easy Vegan Frittata

Preparation Time: 10 minutes Cooking time: 10 minutes

Servings: 3

Ingredients:

½ vegan sausage, sliced

2 tablespoons flax meal mixed with

3 tablespoons water

4 cherry tomatoes, halved

1 tablespoon parsley, chopped

1 tablespoon olive oil

Salt and black pepper to the taste

Directions:

Put oil, tomatoes and vegan sausage in your air fryer's pan, preheat at 360 degrees F and bake for 5 minutes. Add flax meal, parsley, salt and pepper, toss, spread in the pan, cover and cook at 360 degrees F for 5 minutes more. Slice, divide between plates and serve. Enjoy!

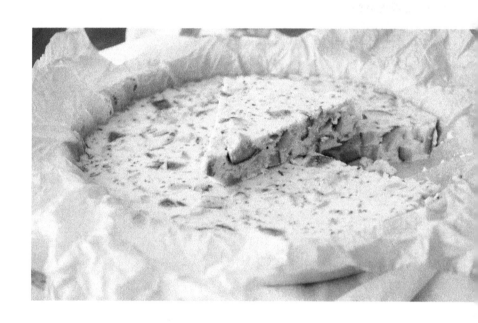

Chinese Breakfast Bowls

Preparation Time: 10 minutes Cooking time: 15 minutes

Servings: 4

Ingredients:

12 ounces firm tofu, cubed

3 tablespoons maple syrup

¼ cup coconut aminos

2 tablespoons sesame oil

2 tablespoons lime juice

1 pound fresh romanesco, roughly chopped

3 carrots, chopped

1 red bell pepper, chopped

8 ounces spinach, torn

2 cup red quinoa, cooked

Directions:

In a bowl, mix tofu cubes with oil, maple syrup, coconut aminos and lime juice, toss, transfer everything to your air fryer and cook at 370 degrees F for 15 minutes, shaking often. Add romanesco, carrots, spinach, bell pepper and quinoa, toss, divide into bowls and serve. Enjoy!

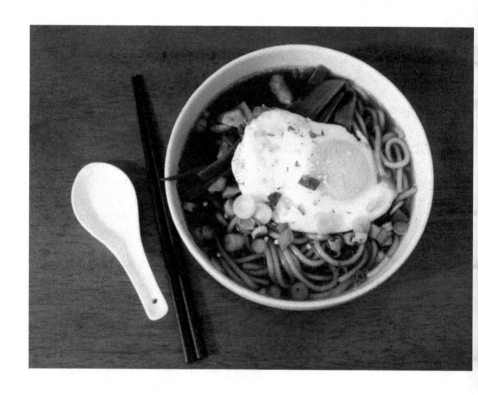

Breakfast Beans Burrito

Preparation Time: 10 minutes Cooking time: 10 minutes
Servings: 2

Ingredients:

2 cups baked black beans

Cooking spray

½ red bell pepper, sliced

1 small avocado, peeled, pitted and sliced

2 tablespoons vegan salsa

Salt and black pepper to the taste

1/8 cup cashew cheese, grated

Vegan tortillas for serving

Directions:

Grease your air fryer with the cooking spray, add black beans, bell pepper, salsa, salt and pepper, cover and cook at 400 degrees F for 6 minutes. Arrange tortillas on a working surface, divide beans mix on each, also add avocado and cashew cheese, roll burritos, put them in your air fryer, cover and cook at 300 degrees F for 3 minutes more. Divide burritos between plates and serve for breakfast. Enjoy!

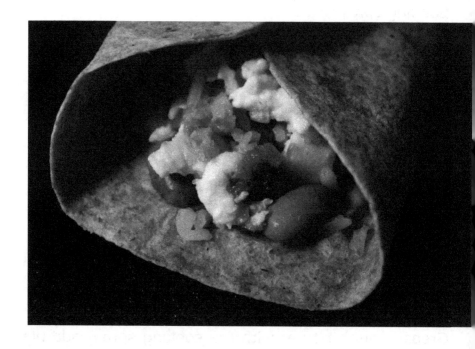

Cinnamon Toast

Preparation Time: 10 minutes Cooking time: 5 minutes

Servings: 6

Ingredients:

A drizzle of vegetable oil

12 vegan bread slices

½ cup coconut sugar

A pinch of black pepper

1 and ½ teaspoons vanilla extract

1 and ½ teaspoons cinnamon powder

Directions:

In a bowl, mix oil with cinnamon, sugar, vanilla and a pinch of pepper and stir well. Spread this over bread slices, put them in your air fryer, cook at 400 degrees F for 5 minutes, divide them between plates and serve for breakfast Enjoy!

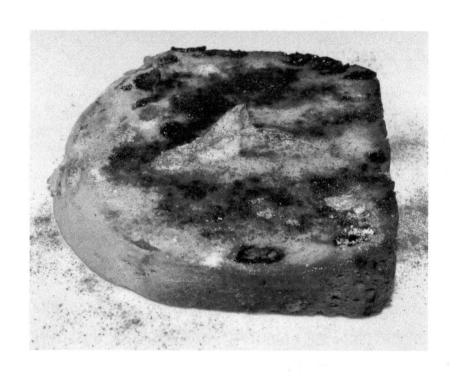

Vegan Granola

Preparation Time: 10 minutes Cooking time: 6 minutes
Servings: 6

Ingredients

2 teaspoons nutmeg

2 teaspoons cinnamon

¼ cup hemp hearts

½ cup coconut flakes

½ cup walnuts

2 teaspoons vanilla extract

1/3 cup coconut oil

1½ cups almond flour

Sea salt, to taste

Directions:

Preheat the oven to about 275 degrees Fahrenheit. In a large bowl, combine all the above Ingredients and mix well. You can melt the coconut oil before adding to the other Ingredients. Spread this mixture in a flat layer on a well-greased baking sheet and bake for about 40-50 minutes, or until the mixture has been toasted. Continue to mix after every 10 minutes, so that the contents can be fully and evenly baked. Remove the baked granola from the oven and let it cool for a few minutes. Store the granola in an airtight plastic container. When serving, serve with almond milk.

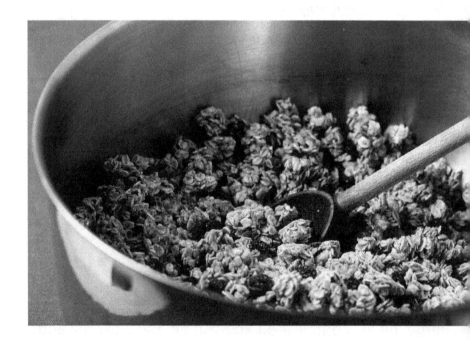

Breakfast Shake

Preparation Time: 10 minutes Cooking time: 6 minutes
Servings: 1

Ingredients

1/4 teaspoon pure vanilla extract Chai tea bag

1/2 teaspoon cinnamon

1/2 teaspoon ginger, powdered

1 cup coconut milk

1 frozen very ripe banana Sweetener, optional

Directions:

Start by brewing the milk along with a chai tea bag. Let the brewed drink cool down fully before blending. Now add in the milk along with the other Ingredients in a blender: vanilla extract, cinnamon, ginger, ripe and frozen banana and sweetener. Process until smooth then serve. Store the remaining in a jar in the freezer.

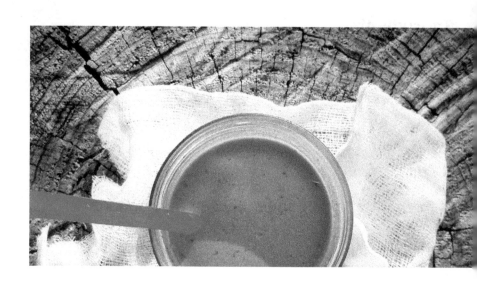

Tasty Vegan Breakfast

Preparation Time: 10 minutes Cooking time: 6 minutes

Servings: 2

Ingredients

Black pepper

Himalayan salt

Juice of 1/2 lemon Flax oil

1 avocado

1 handful of broccoli florets

1/2 capsicum

2 large tomatoes or 12 cherry tomatoes

1 big handful of kale leaves

1 big handful of spinach leaves

50g uncooked quinoa

Directions:

Rinse the 1/2 cup of quinoa and then put the quinoa in a pan with ¾ cup of water. Bring the mixture to a boil and then set the heat to low for the quinoa to simmer while covered. Once done, the quinoa should develop a little curly tail and the water should evaporate. Allow it cool down for a few minutes and then start to steam broccoli for 5 minutes to make it crunchy. Slice the avocados into cubes alongside the kales and spinach. Slice the capsicum and halve the cherry tomatoes. If using cashews or almonds, also slice them up roughly or alternatively bash them with the flat side of a knife. After broccoli and quinoa are done, pour this in a large bowl and drizzle with lemon juice and olive oil. Serve the breakfast and put the leftovers in the fridge for the next day.

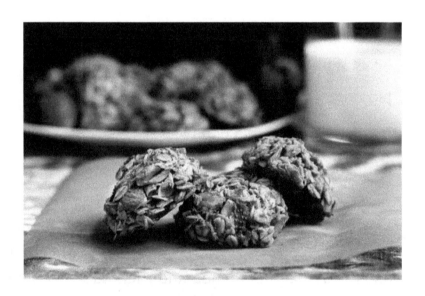

Breakfast Smoothie

Preparation Time: 10 minutes Cooking time: 6 minutes
Servings: 2

Ingredients

1 handful baby spinach

1 cucumber

1/2 avocado

Handful chia seeds

Handful organic oats

Handful cashews

Handful almonds

1 tablespoon coconut oil

200ml filtered water

250ml coconut milk

Optional: 25-50g of cooked kidney beans

Directions:

Put the chia seeds and the liquids into a blender and then process the mixture for about 2 minutes to soften the chia seeds. Once the chia seeds are gelatinous, add the other Ingredients and continue to process until smooth. If you do not have a powerful blender, consider soaking the cashews and almonds overnight to soften them. Serve and enjoy and refrigerate the leftovers.

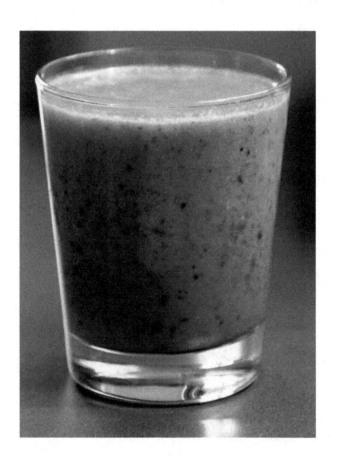

Low-Carb Breakfast "Couscous"

Preparation Time: 10 minutes Cooking Time: 2 minutes

Servings: 4

Ingredients:

200 grams Cauliflower, riced

30 grams Strawberries

20 grams Almonds

20 grams Flax Seeds

60 grams Mandarin Segments

1 cup Coconut Milk

1 tbsp. Erythritol

¼ tsp. Cinnamon Powder

3 tbsp. Rose Water

Directions:

Combine all Ingredients in a microwave safe bowl. Cook for 2 minutes at 30-second intervals.

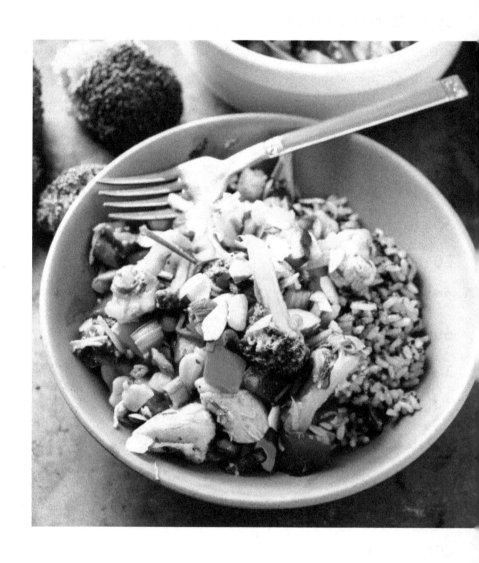

Vegan Breakfast Muffins

Preparation Time: 5 min Cooking Time: 3 min Servings: 3

Ingredients:

2 tbsp Almond Flour

½ tsp Baking Powder

½ tsp Salt

2 tbsp Ground Flax Seeds

¼ cup Coconut Milk

3 tbsp Avocado Oil

Directions:

Whisk together almond flour, ground flax, baking powder, and salt in a bowl. Stir in coconut milk Heat avocado oil in a nonstick pan. Ladle in the batter and cook for 2-3 minutes per side.

Tomato Frittata

Preparation Time: 10 minutes Cooking time: 30 minutes

Servings: 2

Ingredients:

2 tablespoons flax meal mixed with

3 tablespoons water

½ cup cashew cheese, shredded

2 tablespoons yellow onion, chopped

Salt and black pepper to the taste

¼ cup coconut milk

¼ cup tomatoes, chopped

Directions:

In a bowl, mix flax meal with milk, cheese, salt, pepper, onion and tomatoes, stir well, pour this into your air fryer's pan, cover and cook at 340 degrees F for 30 minutes. Divide frittata between plates and serve for breakfast. Enjoy!

Yam Breakfast Mix

Preparation Time: 10 minutes Cooking time: 8 minutes

Servings: 4

Ingredients:

16 ounces canned candied yams, drained

½ teaspoon cinnamon powder

¼ teaspoon allspice, ground

½ cup coconut sugar

1 tablespoon flax meal mixed with

2 tablespoons water

2 tablespoons coconut cream

½ cup maple syrup

Cooking spray

Directions:

In a bowl, mix yams with cinnamon and all spice, mash with a fork and stir well. Grease your air fryer with cooking spray, preheat it to 400 degrees F and spread yams mix on the bottom. Add sugar, flax meal, coconut cream and maple syrup, stir gently, cover and cook on for 8 minutes. Divide yams mix between plates and serve for breakfast. Enjoy!

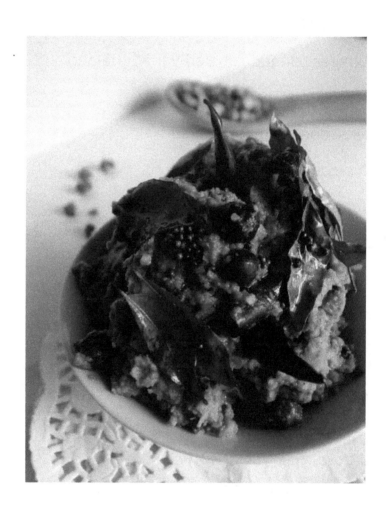

Breakfast Mushroom Cakes

Preparation Time: 2 hours and 10 minutes Cooking time: 8 minutes Servings: 8

Ingredients:

ounces mushrooms, chopped

1 small yellow onion, chopped

Salt and black pepper to the taste

¼ teaspoon nutmeg, ground

2 tablespoons olive oil

1 tablespoon breadcrumbs

14 ounces coconut milk

Directions:

Heat up a pan with half of the oil over medium-high heat, add onion and mushrooms, stir and cook for 3 minutes. Add coconut milk. salt, pepper and nutmeg, stir, take off heat and leave aside for 2 hours. In a bowl, mix the rest of the oil with breadcrumbs and stir well. Take 1 tablespoon mushroom filling, roll in breadcrumbs and put them in your air fryer's basket. Repeat with the rest of the mushroom mix and cook cakes at 400 degrees F for 8 minutes. Divide mushroom cakes between plates and serve them for breakfast. Enjoy!

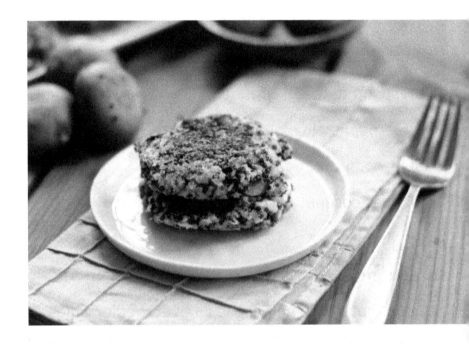

Simple Small Breakfast Peppers

Preparation Time: 10 minutes Cooking time: 8 minutes

Servings: 8

Ingredients:

8 small bell peppers, tops cut off and seeds removed

1 tablespoon olive oil

Salt and black pepper to the taste ounces cashew cheese, cubed

Directions:

In a bowl, mix oil with salt and pepper and whisk. Add cashew cheese cubes and toss to coat. Place a cashew cheese piece in each bell pepper, place them all in your air fryer's basket and cook at 400 degrees F for 8 minutes. Divide peppers between plates and serve them for breakfast. Enjoy!

Miso Oat Porridge

Preparation time: 5 minutes Cooking time: 30 minutes

Servings: 6

Ingredients:

1 Cup Steel Cut Oats

1 Teaspoon Miso Past

1 Tablespoon Tahini

½ Teaspoon Nutritional Yeast

½ Avocado, Peeled

2 Cups Almond Milk

½ Teaspoon Chives, Chopped

Directions:

Mix the tahini, almond milk and nutritional yeast together before placing it in your instant pot. Add in your steel cut oats, and stir. Close the lid and cook on high pressure for four minutes. Allow for a natural pressure release, which will take twenty-five minutes. Mash your avocado, adding your miso paste and chives, and stir until smooth.

Transfer your oats to a bowl and top with the avocado mash before serving.

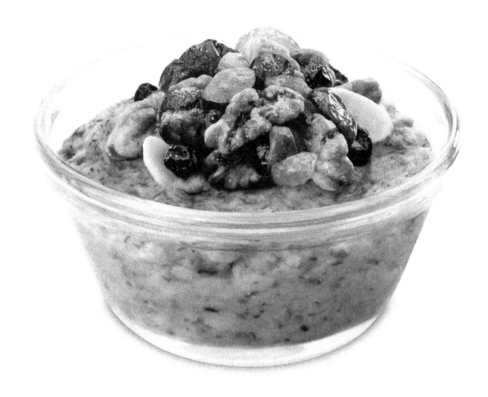

Fig Millet

Preparation time: 5 minutes Cooking time: 40 minutes

Servings: 4

Ingredients:

1/3 Cup Figs, Dried & Chopped

1 ¾ Cup Millet

1 Cup Almond Milk

2 Tablespoons Coconut Milk

2 Cups Water

Directions:

Mix all ingredients together in your instant pot before sealing the lid. Press the soup button, and seal the lid. Allow it to cook for ten minutes, and then use a natural pressure release. Fluff before serving.

Super Vegan Pancakes with Pine Nut-Inspired Maple Syrup

Preparation time: 5 minutes Cooking time: 10 minutes Servings: 3 Pancakes.

Ingredients:

1 cup whole wheat flour

1 cup cornmeal

1 ¾ cup water

1 tsp. salt

2 tsp. baking powder

1 ½ tbsp. olive oil

Syrup Ingredients:

1/3 cup agave syrup

1/3 cup maple syrup

2 tbsp. bourbon

1/3 cup pine nuts

Directions:

Begin by mixing together all of the pancake ingredients in a large bowl. Allow this mixture to sit together for fifteen minutes prior to cooking. Next, oil a skillet and allow it to heat on medium heat. Next, portion about a fourth of the batter onto the skillet, and sauté both sides of the pancake, flipping carefully. Repeat this maneuver with all of the batter. Next, mix together the syrup ingredients and pour this delicious mixture over the pancakes. Enjoy!

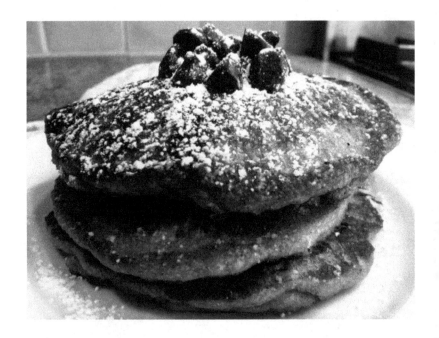

Vibrant Vegetable Tofu Scramble

Preparation time: 5 minutes Cooking time: 30 minutes
Servings: 3

Ingredients:

1 diced onion

1 diced jalapeno pepper

1 chopped zucchini

1 chopped red pepper

1 diced tomato

1 tbsp. olive oil

1 tsp. turmeric

½ tsp. cumin

1 tbsp. nutritional yeast

1 package firm tofu

salt and pepper to taste

Directions:

Begin by pouring olive oil in a skillet and sautéing the jalapeno, the pepper, the zucchini, and the onion for about ten minutes. Next, add the turmeric, the cumin, and the nutritional yeast, stirring well. Pour the diced tomatoes into the mix and continue to stir. After you've completely removed the excess water from the tofu, crumble the tofu into the skillet with your fingers. Stir the scramble together, continuing to break up the mixture well. Salt and pepper the mixture, and enjoy.

Arkansas Apple Oatmeal

Preparation time: 5 minutes Cooking time: 10 minutes
Servings: 1

Ingredients:

½ cup rolled oats

1 tbsp. chia seeds

1 cored and peeled Gala apple

1/3 cup applesauce

1 tsp. cinnamon

1 cup almond milk

½ tsp. ginger

½ tsp. vanilla

1 tbsp. maple syrup

Directions:

Begin by mixing together the oats, the chia seeds, the apple, the almond milk, the cinnamon, the ginger, and the applesauce. Pour this mixture into a saucepan and allow it to heat over medium for ten minutes. After the mixture begins to thicken, take the mixture off the heat and add the syrup and the vanilla. Pour this mixture into a bowl, and add any toppings you desire. Enjoy.

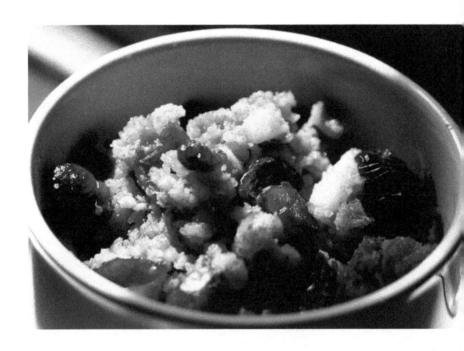

Grown-Up Vegan Chocolate Milk

Preparation time: 5 minutes Cooking time: 10 minutes Servings: 3 cups.

Ingredients:

1/3 cup almonds

2 ½ cups water

1/3 cup maple syrup

1/3 cup cocoa powder

2 tsp. vanilla

Directions:

Begin by placing the water and the almonds together in a blender. Blend the mixture until the water is white and the almonds are meal-like. Next, pour this mixture through a strainer, bringing the created water into a measuring cup. Toss out the almond meal. Next, pour this almond milk back into the blender and add the remaining ingredients. Blend the mixture and continue to alter the ingredients to attain your desired sweetness. Enjoy!

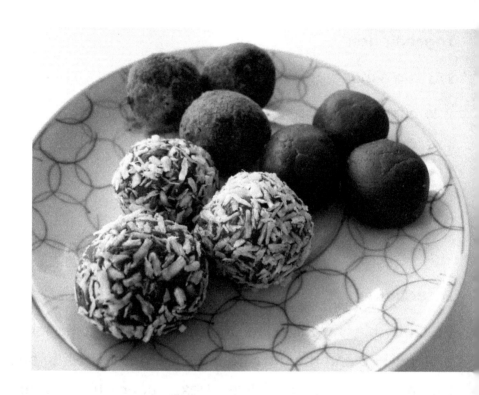

Spinach Artichoke Quiche

Preparation time: 10 minutes Cooking time: 55 minutes

Servings: 4

Ingredients:

14 oz tofu, soft

14 oz of artichokes, chopped

2 cups spinach

½ of a large onion, peeled, chopped

1 lemon, juiced

1 teaspoon minced garlic

¼ teaspoon salt

¼ teaspoon ground black pepper

1 teaspoon dried basil

½ teaspoon turmeric

1 tablespoon coconut oil

1 teaspoon Dijon mustard

½ cup nutritional yeast

2 large tortillas, cut into half

Directions:

Switch on the oven, then set it to 350 degrees F and let it preheat. Take a pie plate, grease it with oil, place tortilla to cover the bottom and sides of the plate and bake for 10 to 15 minutes until baked. Meanwhile, take a large pan, place it over medium heat, add oil and when hot, add onion and cook for 5 minutes. Then add garlic, cook for 1 minute until fragrant, stir in spinach and cook for 4 minutes until the spinach has wilted, set aside when done. Place tofu in a food processor, add all the spices, yeast, and lemon juice and pulse for 2 minutes until smooth. Then add cooked onion mixture and artichokes, blend for 15 to 25 times until combined, and then pour the mixture over crust in the pie plate. Bake quiche for 45 minutes until done, then cut it into wedges and serve.

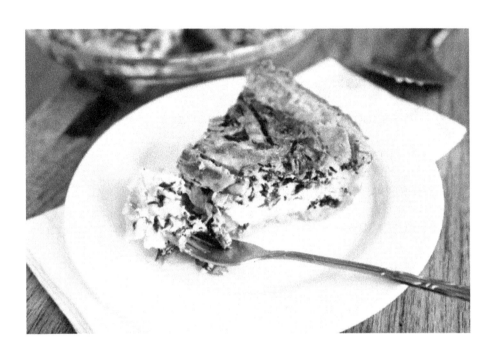

Pumpkin Muffins

Preparation time: 15 minutes Cooking time: 30 minutes
Servings: 9

Ingredients:

2 Tablespoon mashed ripe banana

1.5 flax eggs

1 teaspoon vanilla extract, unsweetened

1/4 cup maple syrup

1/4 cup olive oil

2/3 cup coconut sugar

3/4 cup pumpkin puree

1 1/4 teaspoon pumpkin pie spice

1/4 teaspoon sea salt

1/2 teaspoon ground cinnamon

2 teaspoon baking soda

1/2 cup water

1/2 cup almond meal

1 cup gluten-free flour blend

3/4 cup rolled oats

For the Crumble:

2 Tablespoon chopped pecans

3 1/2 Tablespoon gluten-free flour blend

3 Tablespoon coconut sugar

1/8 teaspoon cinnamon

1/8 teaspoon pumpkin pie spice

1 1/4 Tablespoon coconut oil

Directions:

Switch on the oven, then set it to 350 degrees F and let it preheat. Meanwhile, prepare the muffin batter and for this, place the first seven ingredients in a bowl and whisk until combined. Then whisk in the next five ingredients until mixed and gradually beat in remaining ingredients until incorporated and smooth batter comes together. Prepare crumble, and for this, place all of its ingredients in a bowl and stir until combined. Distribute the batter evenly between ten muffin tins lined with muffin liners, top with prepared crumble, and then bake for 30 minutes until muffins are set and the tops are golden brown.

When done, let muffin cool for 5 minutes, then take them out to cool completely and serve.

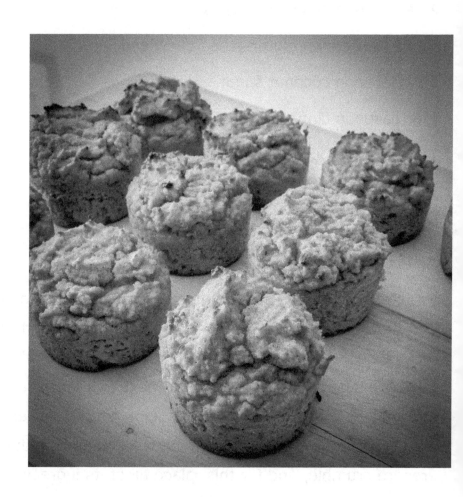

Simple Vegan Breakfast Hash

Preparation time: 10 minutes Cooking time: 25 minutes

Servings: 4

Ingredients:

For The Potatoes:

1 large sweet potato, peeled, diced

3 medium potatoes, peeled, diced

1 tablespoon onion powder

2 teaspoons sea salt

1 tablespoon garlic powder

1 teaspoon ground black pepper

1 teaspoon dried thyme

1/4 cup olive oil

For The Skillet Mixture:

1 medium onion, peeled, diced

5 cloves of garlic, peeled, minced

¼ teaspoon of sea salt

¼ teaspoon ground black pepper

1 teaspoon olive oil

Directions:

Switch on the oven, then set it to 450 degrees F and let it preheat. Meanwhile, take a casserole dish, add all the ingredients for the potatoes, toss until coated, and then cook for 20 minutes until crispy, stirring halfway. Meanwhile, take a skillet pan, place it over medium heat, add oil and when hot, add onion and garlic, season with salt and black pepper and cook for 5 minutes until browned. When potatoes have roasted, add garlic and cooked onion mixture, stir until combined, and serve.

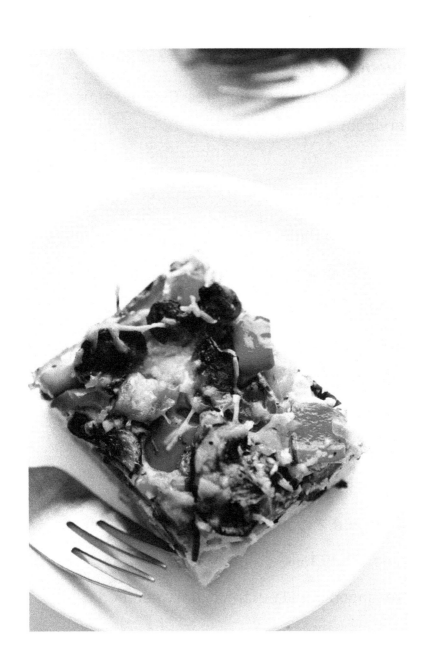

Blueberry Muffins

Preparation time: 5 minutes Cooking time: 15 minutes

Servings: 12

Ingredients:

2 cups fresh blueberries

2 cups all-purpose flour

2½ teaspoons baking powder

½ teaspoon salt

¼ teaspoon baking soda

½ cup and 2 tablespoon sugar

zest of 1 lemon

1 teaspoon apple cider vinegar

¼ cup and 2 tablespoons canola oil

1 cup of soy milk

1 teaspoon vanilla extract, unsweetened

Directions:

Switch on the oven, then set it to 450 degrees F and let it preheat. Meanwhile, take a small bowl, add vinegar and milk, whisk until combined, and let it stand to curdle. Take a large bowl, add flour, salt, baking powder, and soda, and stir until mixed. Whisk in sugar, lemon zest, oil, and vanilla into soy milk mixture, then gradually whisk in flour mixture until incorporated and fold in berries until combined. Take a twelve cups muffin tray, grease them with oil, distribute the prepared batter in them and bake for 25 minutes until done and the tops are browned. Let muffins cool for 5 minutes, then cool them completely and serve.

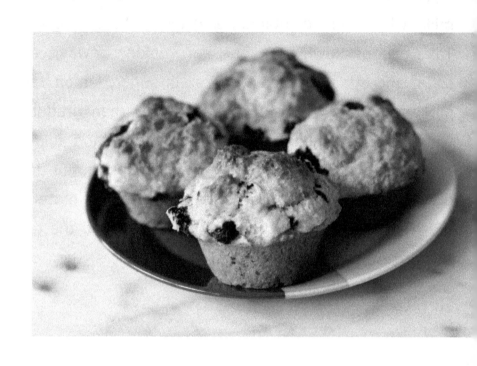

Waffles with Fruits

Preparation time: 10 minutes Cooking time: 20 minutes

Servings: 4

Ingredients:

1 1/4 cup all-purpose flour

2 teaspoon baking powder

3 tablespoon sugar

1/4 teaspoon salt

2 teaspoon vanilla extract, unsweetened

2 tablespoon coconut oil

1 1/4 cup soy milk

Sliced fruits, for topping

Vegan whipping cream, for topping

Directions:

Switch on the waffle maker and let it preheat. Meanwhile, place flour in a bowl, stir in salt, baking powder, and sugar and whisk in whisk in remaining ingredients, except for topping, until incorporated. Ladle the batter into the waffle maker and cook until firm and brown. When done, top waffles with fruits and whipped cream and serve.

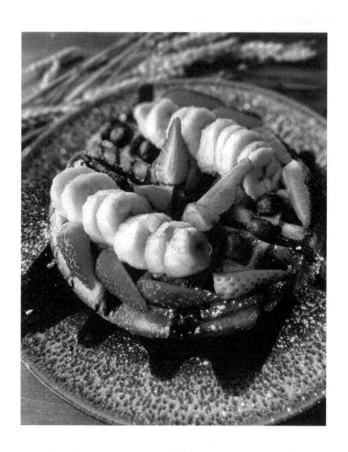

Scrambled Tofu Breakfast Burrito

Preparation time: 15 minutes Cooking time: 20 minutes

Servings: 4

Ingredients:

For the Tofu:

12-ounce tofu, extra-firm, pressed

1/4 cup minced parsley

1 ½ teaspoon minced garlic

1 teaspoon nutritional yeast

1/4 teaspoon sea salt

1/2 teaspoon red chili powder

1/2 teaspoon cumin

1 teaspoon olive oil

1 Tablespoon hummus

For the Vegetables:

5 baby potatoes, chopped

1 medium red bell pepper, sliced

2 cups chopped kale

1/2 teaspoon ground cumin

1/8 teaspoon sea salt

1/2 teaspoon red chili powder

1 teaspoon oil The Rest

4 large tortillas

1 medium avocado, chopped Cilantro as needed

Salsa as needed

Directions:

Switch on the oven, then set it to 400 degrees F and let it preheat. Take a baking sheet, add potato and bell pepper, drizzle with oil, season with all the spices, toss until coated and bake for 15 minutes until tender and nicely browned. Then add kale to the potatoes, cook for 5 minutes, and set aside until required. In the meantime, take a skillet pan, place it over medium heat, add oil and when hot add tofu, crumble it well and cook for 10 minutes until lightly browned. In the meantime, take a small bowl, add hummus and remaining ingredients for the tofu and stir until combined. Add hummus mixture into tofu, stir and cook for 3 minutes, set aside until required. Assemble the burritos and for this, distribute roasted vegetables on the tortilla, top with tofu, avocado, cilantro, and salsa, roll and then serve.

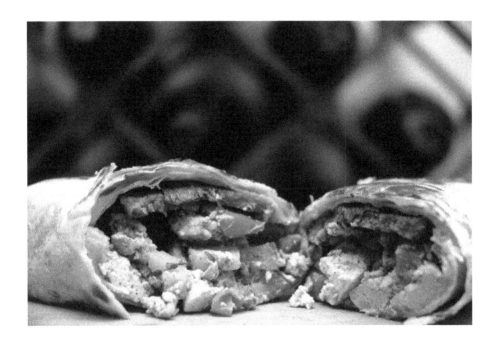

Cream Cheese Waffles

Preparation Time: 5 minutes Cooking Time: 0 minute

Serving: 1

Ingredients:

1 whole-grain waffle

1 tbsp. cream cheese

1 tbsp. granola

1 plum, sliced

Directions:

Toast the waffle. Place it on a plate. Spread the top with cream cheese. Arrange granola and plum, and serve.

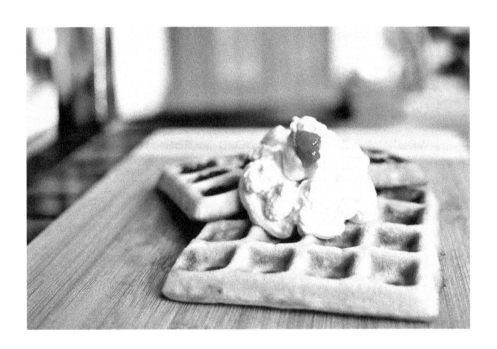

Pineapple Bagel with Cream Cheese

Preparation Time: 10 minutes Cooking Time: 3 minutes

Servings: 8

Ingredients:

8 pineapple slices

4 tsp. brown sugar

4 whole-wheat bagels, sliced in half and toasted

6 oz. cream cheese

3 tbsp. almonds, toasted and sliced

Directions:

Preheat your broiler. Line your baking pan with parchment paper. Place the pineapple slices on the baking pan Sprinkle each with the sugar. Broil the pineapples for 3 minutes. Spread the cream cheese on top of the bagels. Sprinkle almonds on top. Top each bagel with the pineapple slices.

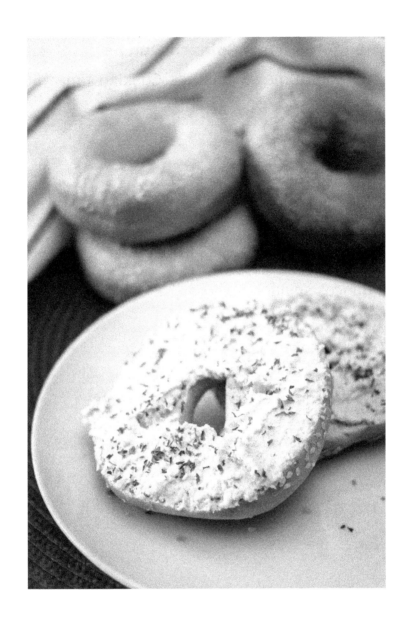

No-Egg Pop Eye's Spinach Quiche

Preparation time: 5 minutes Cooking time: 50 minutes

Servings: 6.

Ingredients:

1 container of tofu

2 minced garlic cloves

10 ounces spinach

1/3 cup soy milk

1/3 cup diced onion

1 cup shredded nondairy cheddar cheese

½ cup shredded nondairy

Swiss cheese

½ tsp. salt

1 vegan pie crust

Directions:

Begin by preheating the oven to 350 degrees Fahrenheit. Next, mix together the soymilk and the tofu in a blender until they're completely smooth. Add the salt and pepper. To the side, mix together the garlic, the spinach, the onion, the "cheddar," the "Swiss," and the created tofu and milk mixture. Stir this mixture well, and pour the mixture into the vegan pie crust Next, bake the quiche for thirty minutes in the preheated oven. Allow the quiche to set for five minutes after baking prior to serving. Enjoy!

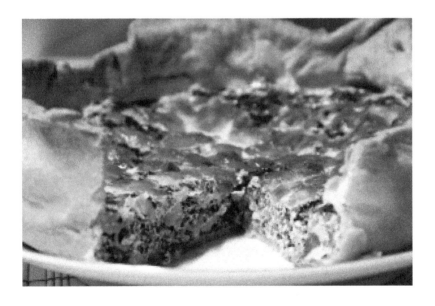

Garlic Flatbreads

Servings: 6 breads Preparation Time: 10 mins Cooking Time: 5 mins

Ingredients:

3 cups plain flour, plus extra for rolling and dusting

1½ tbsp. flax seeds

1 tbsp. instant dried yeast

1 tbsp. sugar

1 tbsp. olive oil

1 cup warm water, plus up to 3 tablespoons more

10-12 garlic cloves

½ tsp. salt Olive oil, to drizzle

Salt and pepper, to taste

Directions:

Combine the flour, instant yeast, flaxseeds, sugar and salt in a large mixing bowl. Drizzle on the olive oil, and then using a wooden spoon mix in 1 cup of water. Sti well to form a smooth dough. Adjust for dryness in the dough by gradually adding up to 3 tablespoons of water Knead for 4 minutes, until the dough is very soft and easy to knead yet not sticky. Adjust for a sticky dough by gradually adding flour, until the correct consistency is reached. Cover and rise for 10 minutes, while you chop up the garlic. Divide the dough into 5-6 equal portions and smooth into dough balls. Roll out the dough, using a rolling pin, until approximately 8-inches in diameter. Heat a large cast iron skillet or large nonstick frying pan on a medium high heat. Simultaneously turn your broiler on to heat up. Place one flatbread in the skillet, drizzle with2 teaspoons of olive oil and spread evenly on the bread while evenly distributing the chopped garlic cloves. Season to taste. After 5 minutes the bottom of the flatbread should be browned, kind of like a properly baked pizza crust. Remove from skillet and place below the broiler, about 3 inches from the top. Keep an eye on the flatbreads and cook until golden and crispy. Repeat until you have six delicious garlic flatbreads. Enjoy!

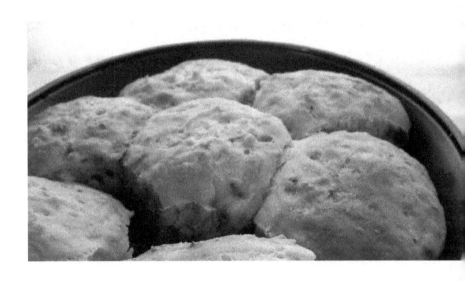

Basic White Bread

Servings: 2 loaves Preparation Time: 20 mins Cooking Time: 25 mins

Ingredients:

4 cups all-purpose flour

1 tbsp. olive oil

1¼ cups lukewarm water

2 tsp. instant yeast

¾ tsp. salt

Directions:

Mix all the Ingredients to make the bread in a large bowl. Using clean hands, knead until a soft dough forms. You may also put all the Ingredients in a bread maker or stand mixer and let the machine knead the dough. Rest covered with a clean and dry kitchen towel, and allow to prove for 90 minutes to 2 hours until it just about doubles in size. Preheat the oven to 480 degrees Fahrenheit. Cut the dough in two equal portions and form the loaves. Carve patterns into the dough with a knife. This will help the bread bake evenly. Bake in the oven until the light and golden. The bread is done if it sounds hollow when tapped on the bottom crust. Recipe Notes: If baking loaves you'll need to bake them for about 20-30 minutes, if making rolls you'll only need 15-20 minutes.

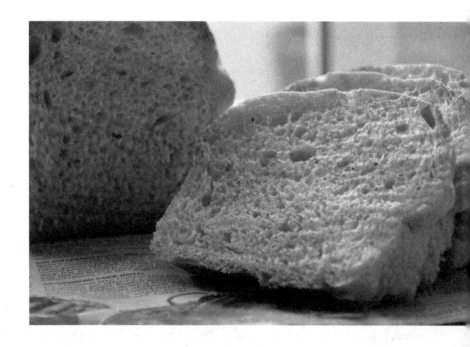

Golden Corn Bread

Servings: 1 loaf Preparation Time: 10 mins Cooking Time: 25 mins

Ingredients:

1 cup all-purpose flour

1 cup corn meal

1 cup almond milk, plus

2 tbsp. more

⅔ cup corn kernels

¼ cup or ½ stick vegan butter or margarine, melted

¼ cup sugar

2 tbsp. golden flax meal

2 tbsp. nutritional yeast flakes

1 tbsp. maple syrup

1½ tsp. apple cider vinegar

1¼ tsp. salt 1 tsp. chili powder

½ tsp. baking soda

½ tsp. non-aluminum baking powder

½ tsp. onion powder

Directions:

Lightly oil a square 8 x 8-inch baking pan and set aside.
Preheat the oven to 375 degrees Fahrenheit. In a
medium bowl whisk together the almond milk, flax mea
and apple cider vinegar. Rest for about 10 minutes so the
mixture begins to curdle. Whisk together the corn meal,
all-purpose flour, baking soda and baking powder in a
large mixing bowl. Then mix the melted vegan butter,
nutritional yeast, sugar, maple syrup, onion powder, chil
powder, and salt. Add the curdled almond milk mixture
Add all the wet Ingredients to the dry and mix unti
smooth. Stir in the corn kernels, make sure that they are
at room temperature and are drained of excess wate
Pour the batter into the baking dish and bake for 25
minutes or until a cake tester inserted comes out clean.

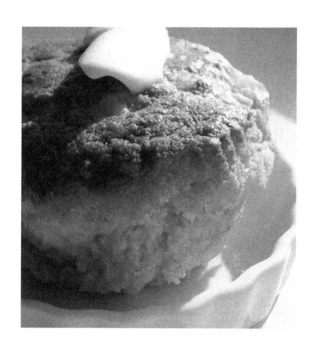

Vegan Variety Poppy Seed Scones

Preparation time: 5 minutes Cooking time: 10 minutes
Servings: 12.

Ingredients:

1 cup white sugar

2 cups flour juice from

1 lemon zest from

1 lemon

4 tsp. baking powder

½ tsp. salt

1 cup Earth balance or vegan butter

2 tbsp. poppy seeds

½ cup soymilk

1/3 cup water

Directions:

Begin by preheating the oven to 400 degrees Fahrenheit. Next, mix together the sugar, the flour, the powder, and the salt in a big mixing bowl. Add the vegan butter to the mixture and cut it up until you create a sand-like mixture. Next, add the lemon juice, the lemon zest, and the poppy seeds. Add the water and the soy milk, and stir the ingredients well. Portion the batter out over a baking sheet in about ¼ cup portions. Allow the scones to bake for fifteen minutes and let them cool before serving. Enjoy.

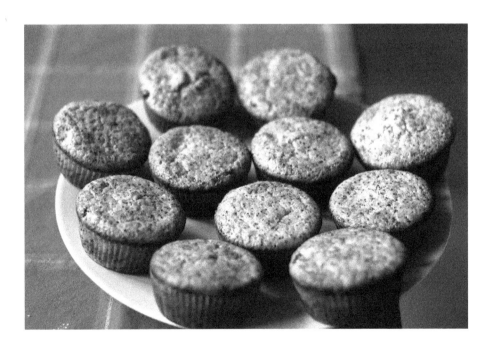

Strawberry & Chocolate Quinoa

Preparation time: 5 minutes Cooking time: 35 minutes
Servings: 2

Ingredients:

2 Tablespoons Maple syrup

½ Cup Water

1 Tablespoon Cocoa Powder, Unsweetened

¼ Teaspoon Sea Salt, Fine

½ Teaspoon Vanilla Extract,

Pure Dash Coconut

Milk + More for Garnish

½ Cup Quinoa

¼ Cup Strawberries, Fresh & Sliced

Directions:

Use a mesh strainer to rinse your quinoa for two minutes
to remove debris. Pour your quinoa into the instant pot
before adding your coconut milk, salt, vanilla, cocoa

powder, maple syrup and water. Close the lid, and then select the rice setting. Set it to low for twelve minutes. Allow for a natural pressure release, and then fluff the quinoa. Add your strawberries before serving.

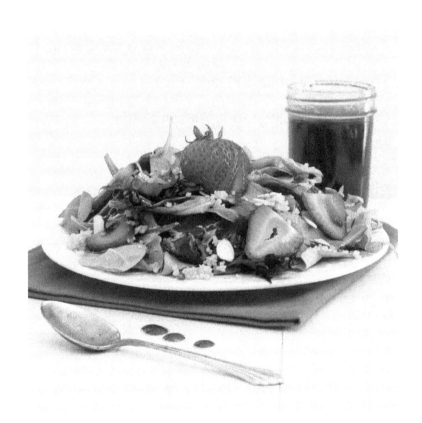

Easy Polenta Porridge

Preparation time: 5 minutes Cooking time: 40 minutes Servings: 4

Ingredients:

3 Tablespoons Maple Syrup + More for Garnish

1 Teaspoon Vanilla Extract, Pure

2 Cups + 3 Tablespoons Almond Milk

½ Cup Polenta, Quick Cooking

1 Cup Water

Directions:

Spray the instant pot down with some olive oil, and then add your two cups of milk, three tablespoons of maple syrup, vanilla extract and polenta in a bowl. Pour in the water, and then put the trivet in the bottom. Place the bowl on top, and then seal the lid. Cook on high pressure for nine minutes before using a quick release. Whisk the polenta until it becomes creamy, and then stir in you milk. Serve warm. It also goes great with fruit mixed in

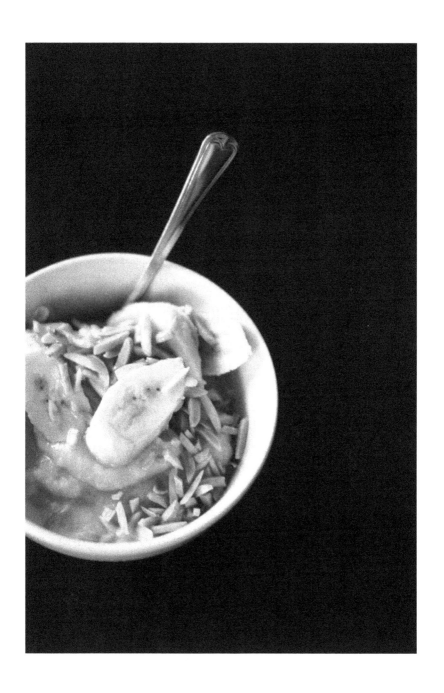

Yogurt Cheese

Preparation time: 5 minutes Cooking time: 40 minutes

Servings: 4

Ingredients:

4 cups full-fat plain yogurt

1 teaspoon unrefined sea salt

extra-virgin olive oil, unfiltered

Directions:

Using a spatula, scrape the yogurt into the lined strainer. Fold the ends of the cheesecloth over the yogurt and refrigerate overnight, or for a minimum of 12 hours. Remove the thickened strained cheese from the cloth. Transfer the mixture to a shallow serving dish and smooth out the top in a circular fashion using a spatula. Make a few swirls in the, then drizzle a fairly generous amount of olive oil in the indentations. Sprinkle with e olives in the middle. Serve with bread for dipping.

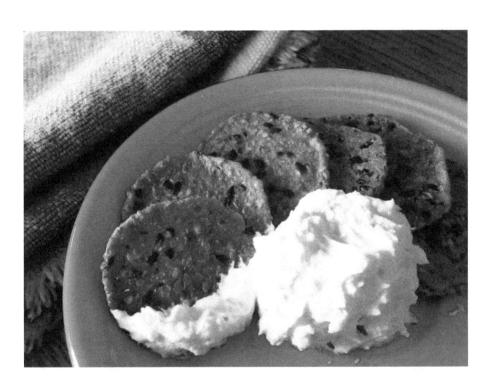

Omelet Provencale

Preparation time: 5 minutes Cooking time: 40 minutes
Servings: 3

Ingredients:

2 teaspoons for serving extra-virgin olive oil

2 zucchini, diced

2 roasted red peppers from a jar, drained, chopped finely
1 clove garlic, chopped finely

¼ cup chives, finely chopped

8 eggs

½ teaspoon unrefined sea salt or salt

¼ teaspoon freshly ground black pepper

½ cup goat cheese

2 tablespoons fresh basil, chopped finely

4 cups mixed field greens such as baby spinach or arugula

1 teaspoon lemon juice

Directions:

Heat 2 tablespoons (30 ml) of the oil in a large skillet over medium heat. Add the zucchini, roasted red pepper, garlic, and chives, then cook gently for about 10 minutes, until softened. Break the eggs into a bowl, whisk lightly and season with salt and pepper. Pour the eggs into the skillet, turn, and swivel to coat. Add knobs of the goat cheese over the top and sprinkle with basil. Slide it back into the pan to cook the other side. To serve, divide 1 cup (25 g) of salad greens onto 4 plates, drizzle with remaining olive oil and lemon juice. Serve a slice of the omelet on the side.

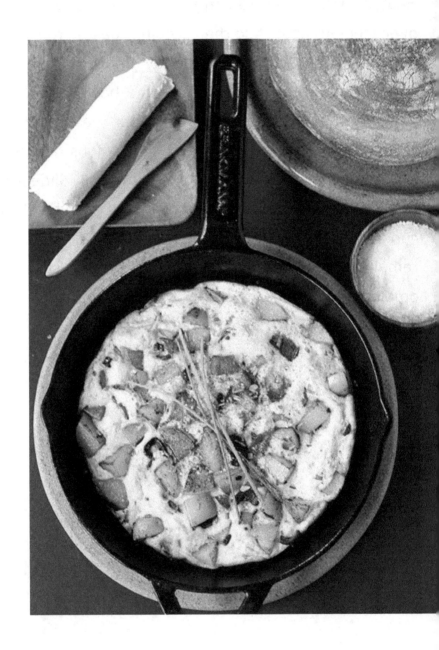

Chili Cheese Omelet

Preparation time: 5 minutes Cooking time: 30 minutes Servings: 3

Ingredients:

2 Tbsp. green chilis, chopped

1 large green onion, chopped

2 tbsp. olive oil

2 oz. Monterey Jack cheese, grated optional garnish sour cream salt pepper to taste

Directions:

Make an individual omelet according to Directions. When the eggs are nearly set, and just moist on top, quickly spread the grated cheese over one side of the omelet. Sprinkle the chopped green onions and green chilis evenly over the cheese and fold the other side of the omelet over the filling. Leave the omelet in the pan, on medium-low heat, for another minute or so, just long enough for the cheese to melt. Slide the omelet onto a warmed plate and serve immediately, garnished with sour cream if desired.

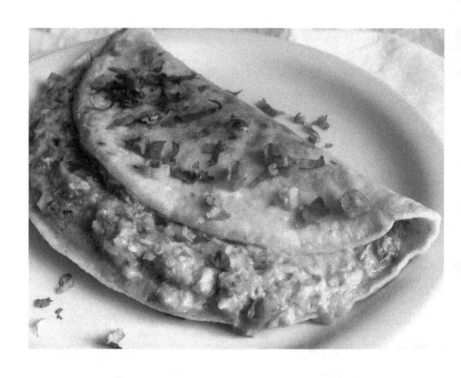

Blackberry Morning Smoothie

Preparation time: 5 minutes Cooking time: 0 minutes 2 servings.

Ingredients:

1 cup almond milk

1 diced banana

½ cubed melon

4 tbsp. wheat germ

½ cup blackberries

5 ice cubes

Directions:

Bring all the above ingredients together in a blender, and blend the ingredients until you reach desired smoothie consistency. Enjoy!

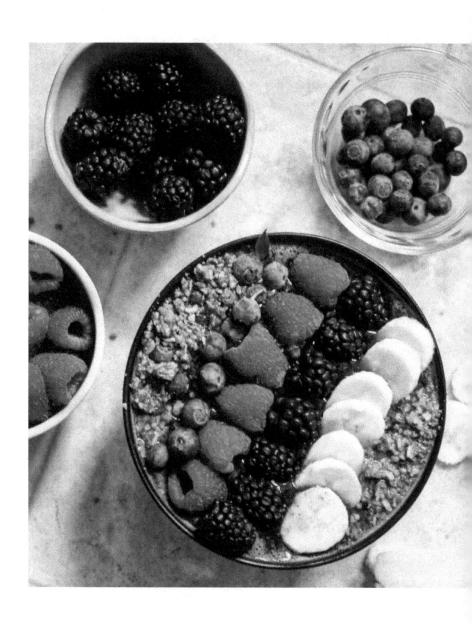

CPSIA information can be obtained
at www.ICGtesting.com
Printed in the USA
BVHW092304250521
608096BV00005B/634

9 781802 696936